I0101588

✎ THE DOCTOR'S GUIDE TO
ALLERGY AVOIDANCE IN THE HOME

Kenneth Wright
In consultation with Dr. Philip Lieberman, Dr. David Rainham

Our special thaks to Physicians Association for Patient Education (PAPE), the American College of Allergy, Asthma and Immunology (ACAAI), the National Institute of Allergy and Infectious Diseases for their members who edited and made suggestions as well as providing established environmental control guidelines to ensure accuracy of the content of this book.

A further thanks to the 32 physicians' offices who allowed the publisher to reference their patient education handouts on environmental control which provided a framework for this book.

Allergies. Home. Patient manual. Allergy avoidance. Environmental control. Self help.

© 2017 MediScript Communications Inc.
ISBN 1-55040-146-7

All rights reserved. No part of this publication may be reproduced, stored in a retrieval system, or transmitted in any form by any means electronic, mechanical, photocopying, recording, or otherwise, without prior permission of MediScript Communications Inc.

Printed in Canada.

IMPORTANT NOTICE

Understanding is your most important tool in coping with your allergy and asthma symptoms. This book can help you in the most fundamental aspect of this health problem: environmental control. This book is not meant to replace medical diagnosis and treatment. If your physician has recommended that you follow some of the suggestions in this book, you should comply. If you are currently under the care of a physician for allergies or asthma, be sure to inform him or her of any changes you make in your environment.

ABOUT THE PRODUCTS & SERVICES IN THIS BOOKLET

The products and services listed are generally accepted as worthwhile by healthcare professionals and, when appropriate, they have been scientifically evaluated. However, there are many other fine products that can help in environmental control that are not listed and that your physician may recommend. It must be emphasized that your physician has no personal interest in promoting these products other than providing you with information to help you control your environment.

SPECIAL THANKS...

...to the more than 30 physicians who allowed us to use their patient education handouts as a resource. Thanks also to the nurses, physicians and allergy/asthma associations for editing and validating this booklet as well as providing the names of reputable manufacturers and service organizations that can help patients. Finally, thanks are in order to the companies and service organizations that provided financial support in the production of this booklet, so that as many patients and caregivers as possible can benefit from this information.

ORDERING

Healthcare professionals who wish to order additional copies or who desire a complete list of titles in the series, please phone: 1-800-773-5088 or fax: 1-800-639-3186, or email mediscript30@yahoo.ca

Visit our website: **www.mediscript.net**

1102007

CONTENTS

PHYSICIAN'S NOTE
You are allergic to the following:

There are other substances that can act as irritants, so I have recommended that you read the sections I have checked to help you manage your condition.

Please read the sections checked on the facing page and take steps to change your environment or take action to reduce your risk, whichever is appropriate.

RECOMMENDED READING

INTRODUCTION

Compared with other diseases, allergies and asthma, for the vast majority of patients, do not pose life-threatening health risks. That's the good news.

On the debit side, however, bouts of sneezing, itching, wheezing, runny nose, and so on can make life miserable. Allergy and asthma victims have good reason to complain of a poorer quality of life. Their main goal is relief of symptoms.

Allergies and asthma are complicated health problems with many causative factors, and each person's ailment is highly individualized. For example, there has been much debate about the definition of asthma.

For our purposes, we'll leave scientific and medical discussions to other books. What we propose to do is to provide some understanding of your environment and some helpful tips to improve your environment.

There is no question that outstanding advances have been made by the scientific and medical communities in the treatment of allergies and asthma. Healthcare companies are producing more effective medications to provide relief of symptoms without causing side effects.

Medical textbooks advocate three primary treatments for sufferers. They are:

- medication
- allergy shots (immunotherapy)
- environmental control

The last treatment is difficult for the physician to enforce. Ideally he/she would have to visit your home, observe, analyze, and recommend. As vital as this appears, it would be an unrealistic use of his or her time. The fact is, though, that home environmental control is common sense coupled with a thorough approach.

You cannot do much about your outside environment, but you can do a great deal to improve the environment of your home. The goal of this booklet is to focus on specific allergens and irritants that can cause problems and to help you create an improved, "purer" home environment. We would like to see you create at least one "unpolluted" room in your home, preferably your bedroom, where you spend a major part of your time.

This booklet is a "how to" approach to achieving these goals. If you follow the guidelines, you will be helping your doctor treat your condition and you probably will find that your quality of life improves.

CHAPTER ONE

ANY QUESTIONS BEFORE WE CLEAN UP THE ENVIRONMENT?

WHAT IS AN ALLERGY?

In simple terms, an allergy is an unusual sensitivity to substances that normally do not affect most people. The dust particles floating around the house that little Johnny breathes have no effect on him. However, after a few hours at home, his sister Jennifer has trouble breathing. She sneezes and develops "allergic shiners," dark rings under her eyes (Fig. 1a). Her problem is caused by house dust.

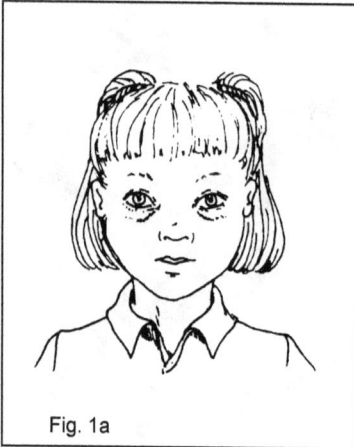

Fig. 1a

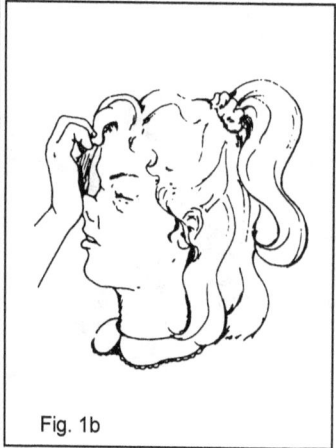

Fig. 1b

You buy a cute puppy for Jennifer the following year, only to find her constantly rubbing her nose, an action called the "allergic salute" (Fig. 1b). This is due to airborne animal dander from the puppy. You now face a major diplomatic dilemma: convince Jennifer to switch to a goldfish!

Whatever the cause(s) of your allergy, the common signs and symptoms are sneezing, itchy and watery eyes, runny and itchy nose, nasal congestion (nasal means pertaining to the nose), postnasal drip (nasal mucus dripping into the back of your throat), and sometimes a cough. Not very pleasant!

A medical term you may have read or heard your healthcare professional use is rhinitis (pronounced rye-night-is). This term covers all the nasal symptoms mentioned, which are caused by inflammation of the tissue lining the nose. When you are allergic only to seasonal grasses, weeds, trees, or flowers, your condition is called seasonal allergic rhinitis.

Jennifer has allergic rhinitis and not seasonal allergic rhinitis, because house dust and dog dander are present all year long.

WHAT CAUSES ALLERGIES?

A quick overview probably is useful here, so that you can understand why you will want to change your environment. The reason some people are allergic and others are not can be found in their immune system.

Immunity is the body's ability to recognize and destroy anything perceived to be harmful. Such enemies are: viruses (eg, colds and chickenpox), bacteria (eg, strep throat, pneumonia), poisons (natural and man-made), and fungi. The normal body produces antibodies that attack and neutralize these enemies.

After these harmful enemies are either inhaled, or swallowed, or touched, the antibody defense system goes into action. In an allergic response specific antibodies latch onto cells in the respiratory tract, or stomach, or intestines, or the skin. These cells are called mast cells or basophils (a type of white blood cell).

The antibodies cause the mast cells to secrete histamine, which neutralizes the offenders. However an excess of histamine creates tissue changes that cause allergy symptoms, such as dilation of the blood vessels, inflammation, and discomfort, which, in turn, cause runny noses, watery eyes, and other annoying symptoms.

In persons with allergies, these antibodies spring into action against substances that normally are harmless: pollen, house dust, animal dander, or molds. So, the house dust Jennifer inhales triggers her immune system to develop antibodies that latch onto cells in her respiratory tract. And, suddenly, the dreaded allergy symptoms are triggered by the release of histamine.

CAN I BE ALLERGIC TO ANYTHING?

In theory, the answer is yes. But, in the majority of cases, most allergies are caused by pollen (from grasses, trees, flowers, and weeds), dust mites, animal dander, molds, insects, or house dust. Other irritants—such as paint fumes, tobacco smoke, hairsprays, perfumes, detergents, weather conditions, even your emotions or exercise—can bring on or trigger allergy-like symptoms.

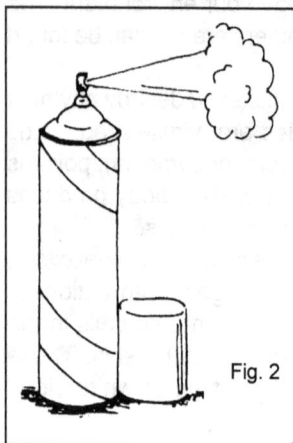

Fig. 2

It is important to understand the difference between these irritants (or triggers) and an allergen that causes a medically distinct allergy. An irritant—eg, an aerosol spray (Fig. 2)—can trigger an allergy-like reaction (runny nose, sneezing, etc.) without being an offending allergen—eg, a weed (Fig. 3). The irritant causes the same allergy symptoms but in a different way. This condition is referred to as nonallergic rhinitis, the most common form of which is called vasomotor rhinitis or VMR.

The question remains: Why does it matter whether your symptoms are due to allergens or irritants? First of all, there may be different treatments for each condition; if you have vasomotor rhinitis (VMR) and not allergic rhinitis or seasonal allergic rhinitis, you may not need an oral medication, just a nasal spray. You actually may suffer from both nonallergic VMR and allergies at the same time. This condition is called mixed rhinitis, and it does not mean that you will feel twice as bad, but it may make a difference in how your physician decides to treat you.

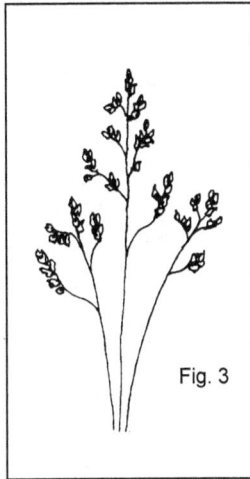

Fig. 3

When you appreciate these medical differences, you realize how important it is to know specifically which irritants/triggers and/or allergens are causing problems. You then can plan to avoid them through removing the irritant and/or allergen, whether paint solvent, mold in the basement, or whatever.

Your physician can complete a comprehensive screening assessment of your susceptibility to irritants and allergens. This can ascertain which kind of rhinitis you have. The self assessment screen is available on the internet at www.AboutRhinitis.com which you can complete and take to your physician if you wish.

WHAT IS ASTHMA?

This question is not easy to answer. For the purpose of this booklet, we will regard asthma as a complex of symptoms involving shortness of breath, wheezing, and coughing. The symptoms are caused by a narrowing of the airways to the lungs. Fortunately, the condition tends to be reversible.

Asthma may or may not be caused by allergens, but most medical authorities accept that often there is a link between asthma and airborne irritants and allergens.

At any rate, we can say with confidence that the preventative measures advocated can do no harm to an asthma sufferer, and there is every reason to believe, on scientific grounds, that the patient will benefit from a cleaner environment.

WHAT IS HAY FEVER?

This term is misleading because there is no fever and the condition is not caused by hay. Essentially, hay fever is the lay term for allergic rhinitis. This condition is characterized by sneezing, with a runny nose, itchy, and possibly swollen, eyes, and sore mouth and throat. The cause usually is airborne pollens from trees, weeds, or grasses.

HOW ARE ALLERGIES DIAGNOSED?

Obviously, there are symptoms we associate with allergies, such as sneezing, runny nose, and watery eyes. The physician recognizes these symptoms as the first clues to a diagnosis of allergy. However, it must be emphasized that other medical problems can cause these same symptoms. This is why it is vitally important to visit your physician to ensure a correct diagnosis, so that treatment can be effective.

The role of the physician in correctly diagnosing an allergy is similar to a Sherlock Holmes approach: a lot of meticulous detective work.

Once the doctor knows your symptoms, he or she will ask a lot of questions to find out the "when, where, how, and what" of the allergy. For example, if you start sneezing and wheezing when the furnace kicks on during the summer months, there's a good chance you are allergic to house dust. If you suddenly start developing watery eyes and sneezing on the arrival of a kitten for your daughter, it is likely that you have developed an allergy to cats, or at least, to cat dander.

Many physicians have their own questionnaire for their patients to complete, so that they can systematically evaluate all of the possibilities.

In addition to the dialogue, completion of a questionnaire, and analysis of symptoms, the physician has some precise and objective ways of confirming the "detective work."

Skin Testing

This is one of the most useful tests for physicians. Drops containing a potential allergen (eg, house dust, pollen, mold, or whatever) are placed on the back or forearm (Fig. 4). The skin is pricked with a needle, allowing the allergen to enter the skin. This is called a *prick* test. A similar technique called a *scratch* test involves making a superficial scratch on the skin and dropping the allergen onto the scratch. In both cases, an area of redness with swelling will develop if the person is allergic to the particular substance. The reaction usually occurs in about 15 minutes. If the reaction is severe, the allergen is wiped off the skin.

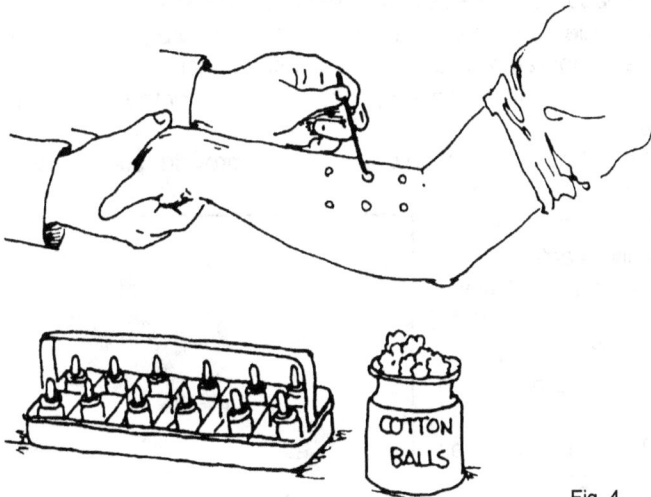

Fig. 4

The intensity of the reaction to the allergen indicates how allergic one is to a substance. These results are used by the physician to confirm the diagnosis. It is possible to have a reaction to a certain allergen but not be clinically allergic to it; this means one may not have symptoms when exposed to the substance.

Blood Tests: A new way to test for allergies

Besides the skin testing, there is a second type of diagnostic testing for allergies which is done on a blood sample. Blood tests are analyzed in the laboratory and are therefore called "in vitro" (in glass) testing.

Although over 400 specific allergens can be tested from blood samples, the physician decides which should be tested. Fig. 5 shows the device in which a complete panel test is performed. The panel, or chamber, consists of 36 preselected allergens common to a specific region.

"Measured" is the key word because this scientific laboratory technique can actually determine, as accurately and precisely as a temperature reading or basketball score, your sensitivity to ragweed, Timothy grass, birch tree pollen or the scallops you may eat.

You may wonder how blood can provide such accurate information about such a simple bodily activity as sneezing when you are exposed to your favorite pollen species from the field next door.

The answer lies in the body's highly developed immune system as explained

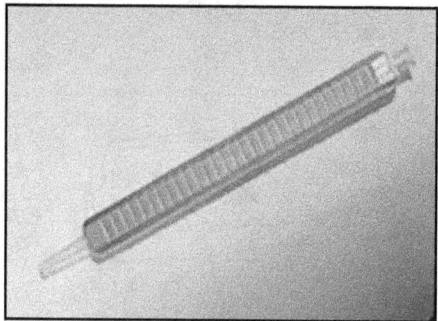

Fig. 5

on page 9, "WHAT CAUSES ALLERGIES".

An allergic person "overreacts" to pollen, dust, etc. and creates more antibodies (these are protein fighters that destroy or neutralize anything foreign that enters the body) in the blood than somebody who's not allergic. If you look upon each allergen as a key—a ragweed key, a house dust key, a cat dander key, a birch tree key—you will see that they are all allergens, but each has a different shape, a different configuration. The miracle of the body's defensive (immune) system is that the blood makes "locks" (antibodies) which can be matched to the "key" allergens.

Laboratories can measure the amount of specific antibody for each allergen present in the blood. This tells your physician exactly how much your body has "overreacted" to each of the specific allergens, from the mold in your bathroom to the dust in your vacuum cleaner.

The name for the allergic antibody is IgE. You'll see this name on your chart and your physician may refer to it. It's just an abbreviation of a complicated technical name. The test that pinpoints which actual allergen could be causing you the problem is the MAST test.

The reality is that hardly anybody is allergic to just one allergen. Therefore, a successful remedy depends on the ability to identify as many of your allergies as possible. This is especially true of the physician's treatment involves "allergy shots" or the avoidance of allergens in your environment, as described in this book.

Physicians use their clinical judgment to choose either skin testing or the blood test to diagnose each patient's allergies—your safety is their primary concern. Your physician can explain about the availability, price, and merits of this procedure as it applies to you in your area.

In conclusion, you have to appreciate that the accurate diagnosis of your allergic condition is very important for planning your most effective treatment plan. The only person that can do this is the physician, by reviewing not just the skin test or blood test, but your entire case history. Drugs can mask symptoms, improvements in the home environment can provide some relief, and allergy shots can help if they catch some of the allergens. Remember, "If you don't know what's wrong, how can you fix it?"

You are probably beginning to suspect that allergies can be a complicated matter and you are absolutely right. So, let's move on.

HOW DO PHYSICIANS TREAT ALLERGIES

Hopefully your physician will have pinpointed what you are specifically allergic to, which can help you take measures to avoid the allergen such as dust, mold or whatever. These environmental control measures are explained within this book. This can help but sometimes you cannot totally eliminate these allergens Also, pollen from plants, trees, weeds are all pervasive in the outdoors and it is difficult avoid these allergens, unless you stay in a controlled environment indoors. Consequently, in most cases, you will probably need treatment from your physician.

Each person's allergy is different depending upon the type, intensity and patient sensitivity. The physician also has to consider possible adverse effects of treatment, possible patient inconvenience, discomfort and cost.

There Are Three Major Treatment Options

☞ Avoidance of allergens and irritants (the focus of this booklet)

☞ Immunotherapy, commonly known as "allergy shots", a series of increasing doses (by injection) of the offending allergen (e.g. house dust, pollen or whatever) to increase resistance to these allergens. Immunotherapy is rather like being vaccinated for polio or chicken pox.

☞ Use of medication, the most common being oral antihistamines which effectively reduce allergy symptoms caused by pollens, molds, house dust or other allergens.

They work by blocking the action of excess histamine produced by the body's immune system, which is trying to fight off these invading allergens.

These products have been approved and used for quite some time and there have been significant advances over the years. For example, the first antihistamines introduced, such as Chlortripolon® and Benadryl®, only brought up to six hours of relief and often caused undesirable side effects like drowsiness. The more recent antihistamines like Claritin, Reactine, Allegra, Aerius, are more convenient to use and have less sedating side effects. During the summer season these medications can dramatically improve an allergy sufferer's quality of life and are available now from pharmacies without a prescription.

The brand leader of antihistamines, Claritin® is now available as a more economical private label brand in pharmacy chains, saving you money without taking away the quality and effectiveness of the medication.

There are other medication options like nasal decongestants (oral and topical) and nasal sprays (antihistamines and steroids). You should always check with your pharmacist or physician to determine what is right for you.

There are natural medicines that can help prevent histamine release and complement your medication. Your pharmacist can advise you on how to mix these safely.

Stinging Nettle: Freeze dried, showed effectiveness in relieving allergy symptoms like itching, watery eyes and runny nose.
Grape Seed Extract: Studies report this prevents the release of histamine.
Quercetin: Known to block the release of antihistamine, reducing the need for high doses of antihistamine.
Vitamins C and E: Allergies stress the immune system and an extra intake of these vitamins can help.
Vitamin B2 (Riboflavin): Use of antihistamines can deplete

Vitamin B2 and cause a sore mouth and tongue. Vitamin B2 supplements can help.

Herbs to avoid
The following have been known to provoke an allergic reaction: Aniseed, Apricot, Amica, Artichoke, Chamomile, Cinnamon, Cornsilk, Cowslip, Dandelion, Feverfew, Garlic, Hops, Hydrangea and Meadowsweet.

Finally: consider palliative, salt based, nasal rinses which can wash away mucus, allergy-causing particles and irritants, thereby reducing the inflammation of the mucous membrane. This helps fight allergies and reduces symptoms.

CHAPTER TWO

FOR THE RECORD

YOUR ENVIRONMENTAL SURVEY

Your physician will ask you some of the following questions. Your answers will reveal problem areas in your environment. We have listed these questions with the rationale for each. Check those that may pose a problem.

Do you live in a city or in a rural area? ❏

In an urban environment, you are more vulnerable to industrial air pollution, which can trigger allergy attacks. On the other hand, living in a rural area may predispose you to high concentrations of pollen that can exacerbate your allergy. Either situation calls for preventative action.

How old is your house? ❏

The older your house, the more likelihood of the presence of dust, mold, fumes, and so on. There usually are more "nooks and crannies" in older houses, encouraging greater dust accumulation. Construction materials also can create problems for allergy sufferers.

What type of flooring does it have? ❏

Hardwood or linoleum floors are best for the allergy sufferer. Older carpets can be an enormous reservoir of allergens: dust, breakdown of carpet fibers, insects, food, and other waste materials.

Are some rooms damp or musty? ❏

Dampness can lead to rampant mold and/or mildew formation as well as possible insect infestation.

What type of heating? ❏

Conventional furnaces without regular cleaning as well as air filter and duct maintenance are a source of circulating dust, animal dander, and pollen. (Do you find yourself sneezing when the furnace starts up? House dust may be the causative agent.)

What type and how old are the window treatments? ❏

The same holds true here as for carpeting. The older the window coverings, the more problematic. Certain materials are better than others. Blinds act as dust catchers.

(Is this questionnaire starting to overwhelm you? Later on, there are succinct checklists on environmental factors; it is surprising how quickly you can make things better with some planning and the services of a few experts.)

Are the bedrooms cluttered? ❏

This is one of the most important aspects of environmental control. You spend much of your life in this room. If you can "purify" the environment here, the benefits are enormous. Eight hours in a cleaner atmosphere gives the lungs, immune system, and entire respiratory tract a chance to build up resistance and meet the outside world with increased resilience.

How old are the mattresses? ❏

This is part of bedroom assessment, but it is worth special mention. Among the most powerful offending allergens is a minute bug one cannot detect with the naked eye. It is called the house dust mite. These repulsive-looking insects feed on dead skin that we shed daily. They are in plentiful supply in mattress covers. It is important to note that they do not bite but simply subsist on shed skin cells. Their excrement and decomposed bodies (disgusting, isn't it?) are extremely powerful allergens. If you notice that you sneeze or have the sniffles when you first lie down on your bed, it's probable that this reaction is caused by the dust mite debris becoming airborne. There are methods for handling this problem: special mattress covers, and wiping down the mattress.

What about hobbies? ❏

Glue fumes, wood dust, the list of possible irritants is endless. These can create problems for you and family members.

Do you have pets? ❏

Even neighbors' pets can trigger reactions, so consideration of this factor is important.

Do you have indoor plants? ❏

Plants can be a source of molds and/or insects. Check them for infestation. Remove them, if necessary.

Do you have upholstered furniture? ❏

"Stuffed" chairs, sofas, and so on are significant dust catchers and often harbor dust mites and other debris.

This is a sampling of the kind of questions your physician may ask you. His/her questioning will depend on your symptoms and when and where they occur. It is hoped that this section has given you insights into the detective work your physician applies in diagnosing your allergies.

A useful aid for your doctor and for you would be a complete record of your allergy problems. This record could be kept for several months or even for a year, or it could be for one week of intense symptoms.

IS ENVIRONMENTAL CONTROL COSTLY?

If money were no object, the ultimate goal would be a house designed to be one hundred percent allergy free! In fact, you can dramatically improve your environment by following some simple guidelines along with, perhaps, the purchase of an appropriate mechanical device. The keys to successful environmental control are *planning, thoroughness in making the changes, and disciplined maintenance.*

SYMPTOM ASSOCIATION DIARY

Back to the "Sherlock Holmes" approach. Complete the Symptom Association Diary at the back of the book for a week, a month, or a year. Record your symptoms, where they occurred, and what you were doing when you experienced them. What was the weather like? Did you notice odors or smells? Record what you suspect the cause(s) of the attack was (were) but remember that the cause(s) or trigger(s) should be confirmed by your physician.

Living with allergies often is a lifelong challenge. We know some allergies are seasonal, which is why it may be appropriate to record your symptoms for a year. Your physician may ask you to complete this diary (or something similar to it) to aid in pinpointing the cause(s) of your symptoms.

CHAPTER THREE

HOME, SWEET HOME

Regardless of your allergic or asthmatic condition, there are certain fundamental preventative measures you should take to minimize your exposure to allergens and irritants. We are not advocating major changes in your lifestyle or buying expensive air-cleaning devices. First, determine how your symptoms are improving before moving on to more sophisticated measures.

Check off each of the following measures as you address them. Remember, thoroughness is the key to an improved environment. It must be emphasized that the measures listed below are "ruthless" but rational actions that are bound to dramatically improve your environment. Compromise will come into play in a number of decisions. The choice is yours. It is suggested that you make decisions that are practical for you.

Pets should not be kept indoors. ❏

This is one of the most heart-wrenching dilemmas associated with allergies. If a person is allergic to a cat, dog, or other house pet, avoidance is the answer. Animal dander—particles of hair and skin—remain in carpets, upholstered furniture, and house dust for many months. So, even if you remove the animal from the home, you may still suffer allergy symptoms.

Get rid of house plants. ❏

Plants may be responsible for the growth of molds, and they can increase the amount of house dust.

Allergic individuals should not be present during house cleaning.   ❑

This is vital to avoid an allergy or asthma attack. If the person must be present, or must carry out the task, an appropriate mask should be worn. Your local pharmacy usually stocks these masks and can advise you what to buy.

Avoid "over-stuffed" furniture.   ❑

If you do own these "offenders," do not sit on them.

Eliminate dust catchers.   ❑

There are too many to mention. Just remember that all items in your home with surface areas that can attract dust—whether shelves filled with ornaments or books lying on counters—should be removed. The principle to follow: AVOID CLUTTER.

☞ **Closets:** Keep them as neat as possible, with everything compartmentalized in boxes, garment bags, and so on. Do not keep what you no longer wear or use.

☞ **Clothing:** Hang clothing in zippered garment bags. Store items like shoes, sweaters, and sportswear in boxes to reduce surface areas that hold dust.

☞ **Clutter:** Remove all clutter: books, boxes, wallets, magazines, papers—anything that is lying around.

☞ **Shelves:** Keep shelving to a minimum. Shelves are among the biggest dust catchers.

☞ **Pictures:** These also collect dust and should be kept to a minimum.

☞ **Ornaments:** More dust catchers. They should be kept in display cases with glass doors.

Carpets ❑

Old carpets create a lot of dust due to breakdown of their fibers. One solution is to remove all carpets and replace them with tiled or wood floors. If you intend to keep your carpets, or they are new, there are ways to keep them clean and relatively allergen free. Professional carpet cleaning can reduce allergens. Or, you can apply solutions that inhibit the formation of airborne dust from carpeting.

Drapes ❑

Sorry! No old drapes, and use only washable window curtains made of a smooth material such as cotton, or polyester, or dacron. Venetian blinds are not recommended because of their dust-catching ability. Roll-up window shades are the ideal solution. Shop around. Many stores are oriented to consumer needs and can provide expert guidance.

Furnaces ❑

Furnaces should be serviced regularly, the ducts cleaned, and appropriate filters installed on the furnace and the vents.

Household products ❑

Avoid products with strong odors, such as deodorizers, mothballs, and insect repellents.

Humidifiers and air conditioners ❑

These should be cleaned regularly because they are a breeding ground for mold spores.

Read Consumer Reports. ❏

Stay informed about environmental control measures. There always are new developments.

Do not allow smoking in the house. ❏

The dangers of tobacco smoke as a cause of respiratory diseases are well known. Passive exposure to tobacco smoke can cause lung disease later in life, especially in children. Tobacco smoke is a powerful irritant that can trigger asthma and/or allergy attacks. If someone in your house smokes and wants to quit, ask your allergist or physician for guidance.

MEASURES TO TAKE: HOUSE

CHAPTER FOUR

THE BEDROOM

Y ou probably spend about a third of your life in the bedroom. It follows, then, that you breathe the air in your bedroom about a third of your life.

If you can clear allergens and irritants from this area, your respiratory system (nose, throat, airways, and lungs) can build up strength and resistance to the barrage of allergens and irritants in areas that are harder to control.

Once you accept that the bedroom should be the focus of your efforts, look at the following guidelines:

☞ Eliminate upholstered chairs, rugs, drapes, and leather furniture.

☞ Floors should be wood or linoleum.

☞ Furniture should be made of wood, plastic, or metal.

☞ Position the bed away from air vents; do not store anything underneath it.

☞ Virtually everything should be washable, including the bedding.

☞ Do not allow pets in the bedroom.

☞ Keep closets neat. Do not store blankets, woolens, sports equipment, and hats in the bedroom closet.

☞ Store clothing in zippered bags.

☞ Use synthetic pillows, preferably dacron or foam. Do not use feather, down, or kapok. Wash pillows monthly. Quilts and sleeping bags also should contain synthetic filling.

☞ Avoid dust-catchers and cluttered surfaces. Keep books, ornaments, and mobiles to a minimum.

☞ If there are vents in the room, cover them with cheese cloth or another appropriate material. If you have baseboard heating, remove the front and sides, so that you can vacuum inside. Dust is a major irritant.

☞ Doors and windows should fit tightly and should be kept closed during pollen and pollution alerts. Keep the windows clean, inside and out.

☞ Clean the room at least twice a week with a damp mop and a damp dust cloth.

☞ Vacuum mattresses frequently and encase them and the pillows in allergy-proof covers with zippers. Replace mattresses every ten years.

☞ Keep children's toys in a box with a lid.

☞ Use synthetic blankets.

☞ Do not use venetian blinds or long drapes. Curtains or shades should be made of a smooth, washable cotton or synthetic. Roll-up shades are preferable.

☞ Installing an air-conditioner can substantially improve air quality.

☞ Keep the decor simple, with as few accessories (including artwork) as possible.

☞ If additional heat is needed, use an electric heater.

☞ Do not use flowers, perfumes, powders, or scented candles.

☞ The walls and ceiling should be washable.

☞ Make it an iron-clad rule that clutter be dramatically reduced or eliminated.

Remember, you and your family probably spend about eight hours a day in the bedroom. The purer the air, the less challenge to the respiratory system and the greater the probability of reduced allergy symptoms. Tick off the items on the checklist as you achieve them. Thoroughness is the key!

IS THIS AN ALLERGY-FREE BEDROOM?

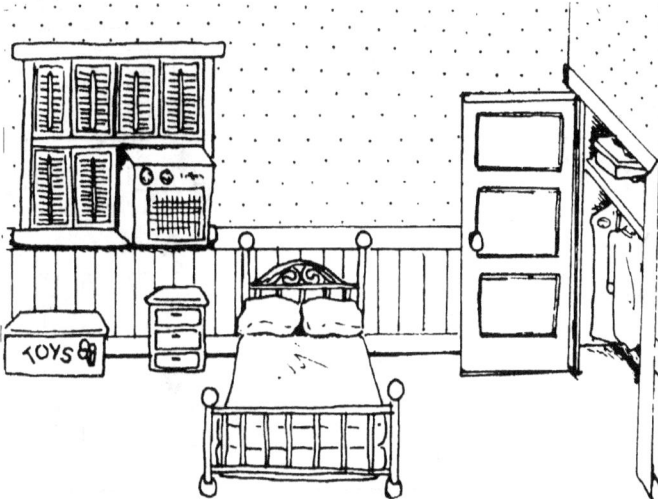

No. There are dust-catching shutters, a closet door open, and clothes are not stored in a zippered vinyl garment bag.

Bedroom Cleaning and Maintenance Guidelines

	Week							
	1	2	3	4	5	6	7	8
Tidy up clutter.	☐	☐	☐	☐	☐	☐	☐	☐
Do not use brooms or dry dusters.	☐	☐	☐	☐	☐	☐	☐	☐
Use water, not sprays, as a cleaner.	☐	☐	☐	☐	☐	☐	☐	☐
Wash walls and ceiling periodically.	☐	☐	☐	☐	☐	☐	☐	☐
Damp mop and dust twice a week.	☐	☐	☐	☐	☐	☐	☐	☐
Clean the windows.	☐	☐	☐	☐	☐	☐	☐	☐
Vacuum nonwashable items.	☐	☐	☐	☐	☐	☐	☐	☐
Vacuum mattress and box spring each time linens are changed.	☐	☐	☐	☐	☐	☐	☐	☐
Wipe mattress covers weekly.	☐	☐	☐	☐	☐	☐	☐	☐
Vacuum carpet at least once a week.	☐	☐	☐	☐	☐	☐	☐	☐
Empty vacuum outside the room. Keep door closed.	☐	☐	☐	☐	☐	☐	☐	☐
If sensitive, wear a face mask.	☐	☐	☐	☐	☐	☐	☐	☐

CHAPTER FIVE

SPECIFIC MEASURES

HOUSE DUST

House dust is a complex mixture of many kinds of airborne particles. You have only to look at a ray of sunlight streaming into a dimly lit room. Eureka! There in front of you is an "allergy airborne division" floating and swirling in the air, causing allergy sufferers to dash for their antihistamines!

The nature of house dust varies from home to home, depending on the character of the house: for example, there may be old carpeting, a family pet, upholstered furniture, decaying insects in nooks or crannies, and so on. These particles can include fibers from carpets and drapes, food remnants, mold, fungi, animal dander, insect parts, debris from furniture, and outside dust. The list is endless.

Check Sources of "Dangerous Dust" listed below and do what you can to eliminate these sources.

Sources of "Dangerous Dust"

☐ Brushes/brooms	☐ Carpeting/rugs	☐ Attic
☐ Vacuum cleaner	☐ Draperies	☐ Basement
☐ Books	☐ Upholstered furniture	☐ Concrete
☐ Chalk/erasers	☐ Toys	☐ Insects
☐ Clutter	☐ Construction site	☐ Pictures

Through testing, your physician may have found that you are allergic to house dust, but it is worth emphasizing that, even if you are not "clinically" allergic to house dust, it still can be an irritant that brings on allergy or asthma symptoms. Consequently, reducing house dust in the home environment is a worthwhile objective.

Dust control in the home should take a comprehensive approach that "leaves no stone unturned."

The measures suggested so far involve minimal cost, but lots of modifications and "elbow grease"! There are, however, other, more costly, measures that involve the purchase of mechanical aids.

In choosing appliances that will benefit your particular situation, you must become an educated consumer. Read, seek the advice of your physician, and shop around. Become an expert!

Chapter Six describes the various home appliances or mechanical devices.

For control of house dust, consider the following:

☞ Centralized vacuum cleaning system or a HEPA vacuum

☞ Quality furnace filter

☞ Air purifier

☞ Periodic cleaning and maintenance of furnace, and especially exchanging or cleaning of the furnace filter.

☞ Consider the professional cleaning of air ducts throughout the home on a regular basis.

Summary of House Dust Control

☞ Complete "Your Environmental Survey," pages 19-22, assessing sources of dust.

☞ Review Chapter Three.

☞ Implement the cleaning and maintenance guidelines in Chapter Four.

☞ Modify your bedroom.

☞ Consider purchasing mechanical devices.

☞ Review Sources of "Dangerous Dust" (page 32), making sure you have done everything you can to eliminate these sources.

MEASURES TO TAKE: DUST

HOUSE DUST MITES

A major component of house dust is a minute creature called the house dust mite. Although technically it is part of house dust, many physicians test for it separately. This allergen requires a separate section regarding measures for its control for several reasons:

- It is a highly allergenic component of house dust
- It is a common aggravator of asthma attacks
- Specific measures can dramatically reduce its numbers
- It is located in easily identified places

The house dust mite is a tiny creature, invisible to the naked eye, preferring warm temperatures (higher than 25° C or 77° F) and high humidity. Consequently the most practical and effective actions to eliminate dust mites are to cool the air by adjusting the thermostat or installing an air conditioner, and reducing the humidity to less than 50% by using a quality dehumidifier.

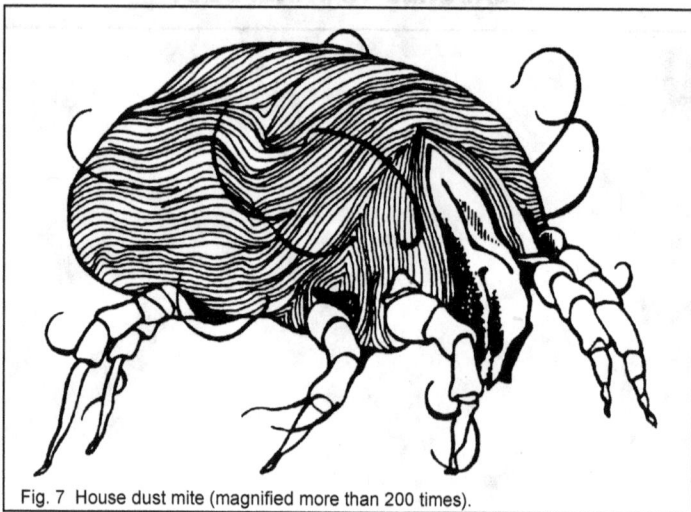

Fig. 7 House dust mite (magnified more than 200 times).

Dust mites do not bite or live on the skin. They subsist on dead skin, which is found on mattresses, pillows, armchairs, carpets, and other furniture. The house dust mite is an allergen because some people are allergic to the decomposition of its body and feces. If you notice yourself sneezing or having an itchy nose when you lie down on your bed, your reaction may be due to airborne dust mite debris.

MEASURES TO TAKE: HOUSE DUST MITES

☞ Encase mattresses and box springs in allergy-barrier zippered covers, and wipe the covers frequently.
Covers vary in comfort, durability, and effectiveness.

☞ Vacuum mattress covers, carpets, and upholstered furniture frequently.

☞ Use a dehumidifier to reduce the relative humidity to less than 50% - aim for 40%

☞ Keep the house cooler, especially the bedrooms.
Air conditioning may be necessary during the summer months.

☞ Shower and shampoo before bedtime.

☞ Consider using a dust mite detection kit that measures how well you are reducing the number of dust mites.

☞ Install a central vacuum system or purchase a HEPA vacuum cleaner to prevent recirculation of dust mites.

☞ Consider sprinkling Arcosan® dust mite powder made by Bissel into the carpet and other high dust mite concentration areas.

Remember, dust mites are part of the house dust problem. All measures that eliminate dust are part of the solution.

MOLDS

Do you feel worse when the weather is damp? Do damp, musty basements bother you? Do you feel miserable if you're near hay, straw, leaves, or a compost pile? If you answered "yes" to any of these questions, you probably are allergic to molds.

Molds are fungi that live off decaying plant life. Molds give off spores that become airborne. When these spores are inhaled by a sensitive person, they produce allergy symptoms.

Molds exist both inside and outside the home. Outside, their spores can be inhaled when one cuts the grass, rakes leaves, hikes in a forest, or does anything outside during warm, humid weather or during hot, dry, windy days.

Inside the home, molds are found in unfinished basements, bathrooms, dried flowers and potted plants, camping equipment, leather goods, stored foods, beer, wine, vinegar, and soy sauce, Molds also thrive in air conditioners, dehumidifiers, and furnace filters that are not cleaned regularly. In essence, molds inhabit damp, warm, dark, poorly ventilated areas.

If you are diagnosed as sensitive to molds, take the following measures.

Dampness

Reducing excessive humidity is the primary goal in controlling mold. If the basement is damp, the mortar may be cracked or defective, there may be cracks in the basement walls, or inadequate drainage. Check rain spouts to be sure that the spouts aren't directing rainwater too close to the foundation. Make sure all drains are in working order.

After you have assessed all the structural issues you can still benefit from the use of an appropriate dehumidifier. Moisture in your home can come from many sources such as outside air, showering, laundry, cooking and so on. Installing a dehumidifier will ensure humidity is kept at a level that does not encourage mold growth.

House dust ❏

Reduce the level of house dust in every room, especially in the bedrooms.

Surface areas ❏

Wash window ledges and shower stalls with Lysol or bleach at least once every two months.

Paint ❏

Use mold-resistant paint for the walls of unfinished basements.

House plants ❏

Eliminate, or keep them to a minimum, or cover the soil with aluminum foil. There are solutions one can add to potting soil that inhibit the growth of molds.

Crawl spaces ❏

Be sure that crawl spaces have adequate drainage to remove standing water. To reduce moisture even more, cover the floor in these spaces with heavy polyethylene sheets.

Filters ❏

Frequently clean furnace filters, air conditioners, dehumidifiers, humidifiers, and vaporizers to prevent the accumulation of mold.

Wallpaper ❏

This is a prime location for mold growth, especially wallpaper in bathrooms. If you do paper bathroom walls, add borax or boric acid to the paste to inhibit the growth of mold.

Damp clothes ❏

Should be laundered and dried immediately to prevent mildew.

Dryers ❏

Must be properly vented to the outdoors to prevent the accumulation of moisture.

Poorly ventilated rooms ❏

Use an electric fan to enhance the circulation of air.

Towels and shower curtains ❏

Expedite the drying process to prevent mildew.

Odds and ends ❏

Papers, old carpeting, old furniture, rags, and so on should be thrown out immediately.

Dehumidifiers ❏

Install and activate a dehumidifier in high-risk areas (such as the basement). Ideally, your goal should be to ensure the optimum relative humidity throughout your home.

Outdoors ❏

Avoid the danger areas listed below if you are sensitive to molds. Remember, molds are found both indoors and outdoors. They are associated with dampness and high humidity. A mold-sensitive person should take measures to eliminate indoor mold and should avoid sources of outdoor mold as much as possible.

Sources of Indoor Mold

☐ Attics
☐ Crawl spaces
☐ Bathroom tiles
☐ Showers
☐ Damp closets
☐ Potted plants
☐ Refrigerator trays
☐ Soiled surfaces
☐ Old bedding and pillows
☐ Stored foods (especially cheese, bread, fruit)
☐ Unfinished or damp basements

Sources of Outdoor Mold

☐ Compost heaps
☐ Hay cutting
☐ Harvesting
☐ Damp garages
☐ Garden sheds
☐ Cottages/cabins
☐ Nature trails
☐ Grass cuttings
☐ Raking leaves
☐ Grain storage
☐ Humid weather

ANIMALS

Although we tend to think of long-haired cats and dogs as the type of pets most likely to cause allergy symptoms, there is no such thing as a "nonallergenic" animal. Animal dander, not hair specifically, causes the problems, and sensitive persons may react to the urine of a guinea pig or the saliva of a dog or cat. Animal dander is a mix of particles of skin, fur, or hair that is shed or secreted and that becomes airborne.

It may be necessary to remove the pet from your home. Even then, since animal dander and feathers linger in carpets, house dust, and air ducts after the pet is gone, it may take three to six months for the allergens to completely disappear.

A good way to determine whether you are not allergic to your pet is if you continue to have severe allergy symptoms after being away from the animal for two or three weeks.

If getting rid of the animal is unthinkable, these measures can help alleviate the problem:

☞ Do not allow the pet in your bedroom. (Remember what was stated earlier about the amount of time spent in the bedroom.)

☞ Keep the animal outside as much as possible Allergy sufferers should not bathe the animal.

☞ Encourage baby-sitters and others who have contact with animals to wear clothes that have not come into contact with the animals.

☞ Professional cleaning of air ducts, carpets, and furniture usually is necessary to completely remove animal dander after the animal has been removed.

☞ There are chemical treatments/ shampoos that you can treat your animal with that can render the dander less allergenic. Allerpet is one well proven brand name. Your veterinarian or pet store can advise you on the products available.

☞ When your pet dies, don't replace it with a different type of animal. Someone allergic to one kind of animal may develop an allergy to the new animal.

☞ If you are going to visit someone who has an animal, take antihistamines or asthma medication and/or have your child take it, so that you and/or your child will be able to tolerate limited exposure to the animal. If you are staying overnight, the animal should be temporarily removed, and the room you sleep in should be thoroughly cleaned and the bedding changed before your visit.

Keep in mind that living animals are not the only source of allergens. Clothing made of mohair, alpaca, cashmere, or goat hair can trigger allergic reactions, as can horsehair-stuffed chairs and couches. Feathers and down can do the same. If you are sensitive to feathers, stay away from comforters, sleeping bags, and ski jackets that are filled with down and/or feathers. Use synthetic-filled items instead. Avoid foam rubber since it encourages the growth of mold.

MEASURES TO TAKE: ANIMALS

POLLEN AVOIDANCE

Pollens are the fertilizing agents of flowering plants, including trees, grasses, and weeds. Different pollens are abundant at different times of the year. Your physician can gather many clues to your sensitivity by asking at which time of the year you are most troubled by allergies. Weeds generally pollinate in the fall, whereas trees and grasses pollinate in the spring.

Pollens are microscopic and capable of being carried through the air for great distances. A good analogy is to regard them as microscopic balloons, invisible to the naked eye, floating in huge masses. Millions, sometimes billions, can be released by one plant. Many colorless, not particularly fragrant plants produce large amounts of pollen because they can not rely on insects that are attracted by colour and fragrance to carry out fertilization.

Ragweed seasons in the United States

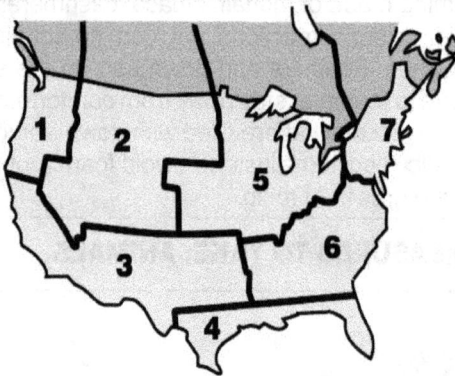

Ragweed season usually lasts four to six weeks. Dates throughout the United States are as follows:

1. July through mid October
2. July through mid August
3. Late July through mid October
4. Mid March through mid October
5. Early August through mid October
6. Mid July through October
7. Early August through mid October

Two windborne grass pollens that pollinate in May and June are shown on the left: Timothy grass and Blue grass. If you are allergic to pollens, determine which plants bother you and their times of pollination. If these plants grow around your house, you may find some relief by eliminating them. But remember, pollen can be airborne for long distances so your chances of complete relief are slim.

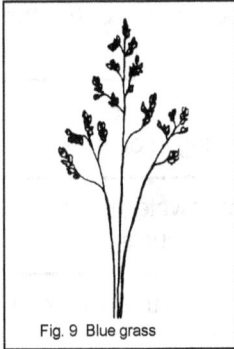

Fig. 8 Timothy grass

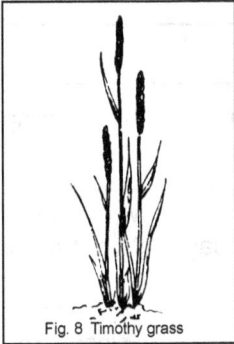

Fig. 9 Blue grass

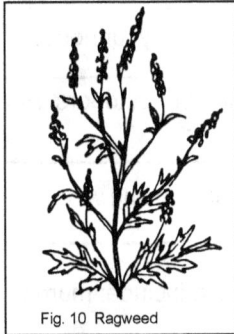

Fig. 10 Ragweed

The most problematic pollen is ragweed (Fig. 10), which prevails August through September. Farther west, ragweed eventually disappears, so if you take your holidays in California, or on the West Coast of Canada or the United States, you may be symptom free!

To appreciate the impact of ragweed, consider this: one ragweed plant can release billions of pollen grains, and these can travel more than 100 miles a day, farther on windy days. In eastern and central Canada and the United States, it is estimated that well over 300 million tons of pollen are circulated August and September.

Because pollen can be carried great distances, you should be aware not only of plants growing in your immediate vicinity but also of those that grow in your county and state.

Weather conditions play their part. Pollen counts are lower in rainy weather, higher in the early morning and during warm, dry weather.

Not all pollens cause reactions. Pine tree pollen, for instance, doesn't seem to be a problem, whereas poplar, beech, and oak pollens are common instigators.

Guidelines for Pollen Avoidance

Pollen poses difficulties in terms of control, but the following guidelines will help:

☞ Avoid, if you can, going outdoors on days when pollen counts are high, namely dry, windy days, late evenings, and early mornings.

☞ Close all windows, especially when you sleep. The allergy sufferer should occupy a cool room, so that the bedroom window(s) can be kept closed.

☞ Air conditioning decreases indoor pollen counts if it recirculates indoor air instead of drawing in outside air.

☞ Fans in the attic or other rooms may aggravate the problem by drawing in outside air with high pollen counts.

☞ Keep car windows closed during trips to the country. If possible, have air conditioning in the car.

☞ Don't plant a lot of trees and shrubs around your house.

☞ Shower and shampoo after coming in from outdoors. Put on fresh clothing after you shower.

☞ Eliminate weeds by uprooting them and/or using weed killers.

☞ Avoid plants related to ragweed. These include: mums, zinnias, dahlias, and sunflowers.

☞ Consider installing an electronic/electrostatic furnace filter and an air purifier.

☞ Check your weather network, newspaper, or national allergy bureau for pollen forecasts (1-800-9-POLLEN).

☞ If you are going to drive and want nondrowsy allergy relief, read the package insert of your allergy medication. If your allergy medication cautions you about driving while under its influence, then it probably is not nondrowsy.

There is little you can do about the outside environment with regard to massive amounts of airborne pollen. You can, however, minimize pollen counts in your home, especially in your bedroom. You will enjoy a better quality of life in your own home if you follow these guidelines.

Medications

Many ragweed and other pollen allergy sufferers would have difficulty functioning without medication, even if they have made improvements to their home environment. The new generation of antihistamines controls the symptoms of sneezing, runny nose, and itchy, watery eyes without causing drowsiness. This enables allergy sufferers to maintain a good quality of life during the pollen season. Corticosteroid nasal sprays are another type of medication that relieves allergy symptoms.

Your physician will determine which type of medication is appropriate for you.

INDOOR AIR POLLUTION

Our homes are filled with cleaning products, bath oils, scented candles, mothballs, insect repellants, and floor wax products. Such items generate odors and fumes that can cause allergy symptoms in sensitive people. Poor ventilation can worsen the problem.

Tobacco smoke is a common indoor air pollutant. Studies have shown that children exposed to tobacco smoke—even with only parent smoking—are more likely to develop respiratory infections, whether or not they have allergies. Children are less likely to develop allergies of any kind if those around them don't smoke. If a smoker ever needed a good reason to quit, having an allergic child would certainly be one.

Natural gas can be a problem for chemically sensitive individuals. Gas-fired furnaces and stoves discharge fumes into the household environment. Consult you local heating engineer for advice.

Of course, some irritants come from outdoors. If you live on or near a busy street, you may have to keep your windows shut during peak traffic hours. If you live near a factory, the smoke may cause problems.

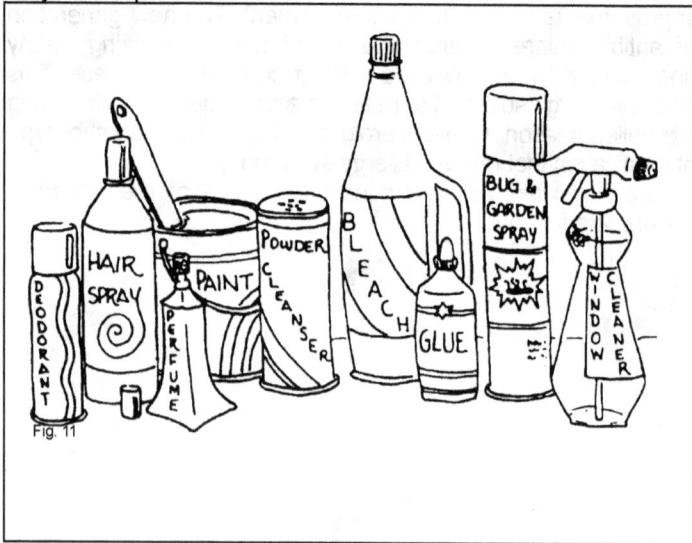

Fig. 11

You may even decide that it is in your best interests to move if prevailing winds carry industrial pollution into your home.

A plethora of fumes, smoke, household aids, and cosmetics may be bothering you. It is important to understand that these are irritants rather than allergens. Nevertheless, they can lower your resistance and irritate your respiratory system, thereby lowering your allergy sensitivity thresholds. Review the following and check the items (on page 61) that you believe to be detrimental to your well-being:

Outside vents from the kitchen, bathroom, and clothes dryer should be located as high as possible, so that exhaust fumes are not recirculated.

If possible, replace natural gas heat and gas appliances with electric hot water heating and electric appliances. If that is not possible, ask your utility company to turn off the pilot light on your stove. (Use matches to light the stove.) Install an exhaust hood above the stove and an air filter in the kitchen to remove cooking odors. Make sure that the exhaust from your gas furnace is going up the chimney rather than escaping into the house or ducts.

If your garage is attached, check the rooms above it and adjacent to it for odors from chemicals stored in the garage.

Keep containers of paints, solvents, insecticides, household cleaning products, glues, and so on tightly sealed.

Items That Can Cause Problems

- Car exhaust
- Furnace
- Kerosene
- Glue
- Ammonia
- Floor waxes
- Perfumes
- Tobacco
- Rubber
- Dry cleaning fluid
- Moth balls
- Swimming pool
- Window cleaners
- Bleaches
- Detergents
- Paint
- Nail polish
- Marking pens
- Gasoline
- Motor oil
- Garages
- Disinfectants
- Deodorants
- Aerosol sprays
- Smoke
- Solvents
- Pungent foods
- Strong odors

MEASURES TO TAKE: INDOOR AIR POLLUTION

CLIMATE AND OUTDOOR AIR POLLUTION

There is no doubt that climate plays an important role in inducing or exacerbating asthma and allergy symptoms. High humidity, sudden temperature changes (especially from warm to cold), and decreases in barometric pressure all have adverse effects on allergy and asthma sufferers. Damp conditions encourage the growth of mold and dust mites.

Families often are advised to move to a more favorable climate, if possible, although there is no hard evidence that such relocations help.

Smog is another factor over which we have little control. In warm, sunny climates (eg, Los Angeles), heavy traffic creates a smog composed mainly of ozone, nitrogen dioxide, and petroleum-produced chemicals called hydrocarbons. Industrial cities produce their particular brand of smog. Whatever its composition, smog causes eye irritation, breathing problems, and fatigue as well as other symptoms.

The following are guidelines for coping with air pollution. They are especially relevant for asthmatics, who tend to be more adversely affected by air pollution and climatic changes.

COPING WITH AIR POLLUTION

☞ Stay indoors in a clean environment as much as possible.

☞ Use air conditioners, air filters, electrostatic furnace filters, or any other device that helps purify the air.

☞ Avoid smoke-filled rooms and exposure to dust and other irritants, such as paint fumes, hair spray, and so on.

☞ Avoid unnecessary physical activity.

☞ If pollution is predicted to worsen and remain severe for a prolonged period, consider leaving the area if circumstances permit doing so.

☞ Keep emergency telephone numbers handy in case of a medical emergency.

☞ Have a face mask available. Pharmacists generally stock them.

The asthmatic is more sensitive to the outside environment. Climatic changes, "the greenhouse effect," and global air pollution are now being taken seriously by our political leaders. We hope that, in this new century, we will see responsible leadership in protecting our precious planet and its inhabitants.

MEASURES TO TAKE: OUTDOOR AIR POLLUTION

CAR

Driving a car, especially with the windows open, exposes driver and occupant to numerous airborne irritants and allergens: pollen, asphalt, tar, fertilizers, car exhaust fumes—the list is long.

COPING WITH CAR TRAVEL

☞ Keep windows closed.

☞ If possible, install air conditioning.

☞ If you have air conditioning, have it serviced (and the ducts cleaned) before you use it after a long lay-off. Otherwise, you may be blasted with dust when you first turn it on. Check with the manufacturer or with your local auto service for a recommended schedule of servicing.

☞ Mold also can grow in auto air-conditioning units, so this is another good reason for regular servicing.

☞ Keep the interior of your car clean: vacuum the carpets, wipe the seats, and so on. The same principles for dust prevention in your house apply to your car.

☞ Filters are now available in many models of cars. You should ensure that you change your filter after the recommended number of miles driven.

COCKROACHES

These ugly creatures do not intend to scare you or to make you sick; they are just looking for food. Eliminating their food sources is the key to eliminating them. Their bodily waste, like that of the house dust mite, can cause allergic reactions. However, the onset of an allergic reaction is somewhat slower than that of other allergens. One has to inhale a significant quantity in an infested area before a reaction occurs.

Cockroaches are a successful species, having remained relatively unchanged for 400 million years. There are more than 3,500 species. However, only eight species are found indoors in North America. Cockroaches are highly adaptable and indigenous to tropical climates. With the advent of centrally-heated homes, they can live anywhere in any season.

It is estimated that more than ten million people in the United States are allergic to cockroaches, and about 40 percent of asthma sufferers are thought to be allergic to cockroaches.

☞ Cockroaches are attracted to food and to warm, moist areas.

Cockroaches are found, in order of magnitude, in:

1. Kitchen cabinets
2. Kitchen floors
3. Damp basements
4. Mattresses
5. Upholstered furniture
6. Bathrooms
7. Soft furnishings
8. Toilets
9. Bedrooms
10. Anywhere there is water and food

Eliminating cockroaches

Getting rid of these pests is your number-one priority. Roach traps can be effective, but if infestation is severe, you may need a commercial exterminator. The best long-term approach is to reduce the attraction of your home, so they leave for "greener pastures." Make it more difficult for cockroaches to enter your home by closing entry points with sealants. Talk to your local hardware store for practical advice. Here's a checklist.

Reduce food sources.

Restrict all eating to the dining room and kitchen. Use trays if eating elsewhere and wash them regularly.

Wash dirty dishes and clean counters immediately. Don't let dirty dishes sit in the dishwasher.

Clean up crumbs and spills immediately. Keep drawers, cabinets, microwaves, ovens, and refrigerators clean. Do not let soil accumulate.

Ensure that all food garbage is tightly sealed in one garbage can and empty the can often. Wash the can regularly.

Don't leave your pet's food out overnight.

Store all dry foods in tightly sealed containers.

Clean drawers regularly. Dispose of "junk."

Regularly throw away (or recycle) paper products (especially those from the grocery store), newspapers, and magazines.

Reduce dampness.

☞ Remove rotted flooring and damp wallpaper.

☞ When painting or wall-papering, make sure fungicide is applied to walls beforehand.

☞ Fix leaking pipes.

☞ Waterproof cement floors in the garage and basement. Cover with plastic to prevent moisture from rising.

☞ Repair cracks in the foundation.

☞ Install dehumidifiers and fans to reduce the moisture level (relative humidity). Aim for 40%; humidity must be below 50% to discourage infestation of cockroaches.

Elimination of cockroach infestation and subsequent prevention of reinfestation are challenges. Thoroughness in reducing food sources and dampness can prevent reinfestation.

MEASURES TO TAKE: COCKROACHES

AVOIDING ANAPHYLAXIS
(severe allergic reaction)

What is Anaphylaxis (pronounced an-uh-fuh-lak-sis)

Anaphylaxis is a potentially life threatening severe allergic reaction that involves the entire body. Some of the symptoms can include itching, dizziness, and more seriously, difficult breathing, loss of consciousness and even death, if not immediately treated.

Anaphylaxis is a medical emergency that requires immediate medical treatment and later follow up care.

Causes or triggers of Anaphylaxis

Obviously it is very important to know what causes your severe allergic reactions in order to be able to avoid the cause. If you are unsure, your physician can do a skin or blood test (see pages 13 – 16) to pinpoint the culprit.

The most common causes or triggers include: food, insect stings, latex and medications. How to avoid these triggers will be explained later in this section.

Occasionally exercise can trigger anaphylaxis and there can be other or unknown causes; this is called idiopathic anaphylaxis.

Anaphylaxis caused by other triggers

Although much less common than insects or food, other triggers include:

Latex in rubber gloves, elastic bands, balloons, condoms and medical supplies.

Medications, especially penicillin, can bring on anaphylaxis. Your physician normally checks for this potential problem.

Recognizing the symptoms

It is important to understand that not all symptoms of anaphylaxis have to be present, symptoms do not appear in any particular order and each person's reaction is unique. The symptoms may begin in as little as five to fifteen minutes to up to two hours after exposure to the allergen, but life threatening reactions may progress over hours.

Common Symptoms

Skin: itching, hives, swelling, flushing of the face or body, tingling or a warm sensation.

Respiratory: throat tightness, chest tightness, wheezing, coughing, difficulty breathing.

Gastrointestinal: stomach cramping, diarrhea, vomiting, difficulty swallowing.

Mental: sense of fear, feeling faint, loss of consciousness (due to low blood pressure).

Taste: a metallic taste in the mouth.

Treatment of Anaphylaxis

The fundamental "emergency" treatment is a self - injection of epinephrine (also known as adrenalin), usually injected into the front of the thigh. The injection immediately helps you breathe by relaxing the narrowed airways in the lung and simultaneously helps increase blood pressure by constricting small blood vessels.

These injections are available by prescription from your physician and it is advisable to carry them with you always in case of such an emergency. It is always advisable to seek medical treatment at a clinic or hospital even after your epinephrine injection. You must also consider that the effects of epinephrine wear off 10 to 20 minutes after injection. Further, it has also been estimated one out of every three people may have a reaction severe enough to require more than one dose of epinephrine.

One epinephrine injection prescribed by physicians is Twinject® which addresses this critical need and provides 2 doses of epinephrine in one device.

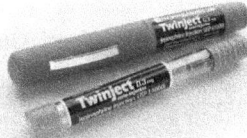

Prevention is better than cure

If you know you are vulnerable to anaphylaxis, it is highly advisable you discuss with your physician the preventative measures you can take like obtaining an epinephrine injection kit, obtaining a MedicAlert® bracelet or necklet, 1 888 904 7629 (this immediately helps any helper or medical person attending you), devising an emergency response plan and considering a series of allergy shots that can provide immunity to anaphylaxis. DO NOT LEAVE ANYTHING TO CHANCE.

Avoiding Anaphylaxis from stinging / biting insects

More than two million North Americans are allergic to stinging insects. The degree of allergy varies widely. Although most are just local reactions around the sting / bite skin site, many, however, will have severe allergic reactions (anaphylaxis). 50 – 150 deaths occur each year from these stings, and up to one million hospital visits result from insect stings. The majority of stinging insects that can cause anaphylaxis are bees, yellow jackets, hornets, wasps and fire ants. The fire ants are only found in the southeastern United States. The following guidelines for avoiding insects are most appropriate during the summer months when insects are highly active.

Avoiding Stinging / Biting Insects

☞ Always wear closed-toe shoes outdoors, avoid going barefoot. Even smooth beach sand can harbor certain types of wasps.

☞ Avoid wearing loose clothing in which insects can become trapped. Choose clothing that covers arms and legs when outside.

☞ Wear light colored clothing. White, green, tan and khaki are least attractive to insects. Insects are attracted to bright colors and floral patterns. Bees find black irritating but blue comforting. Also materials like denim and corduroy attract insects.

☞ Avoid colognes, perfumes, scented lotions, soaps and hairspray.

☞ Avoid the following, especially when gardening, because they often harbor nests of stinging insects: old trees, clover bushes, shrubs, large rocks, logs, woodpiles, eaves of buildings and shutters.

☞ Keep the area around garbage cans clean and spray the cans with insecticide.

☞ Be cautious around bird baths, puddles, and pet bowls where insects like to feed.

☞ Always keep food covered and approach picnic areas cautiously. Leftover food and strong smells attracts insects.

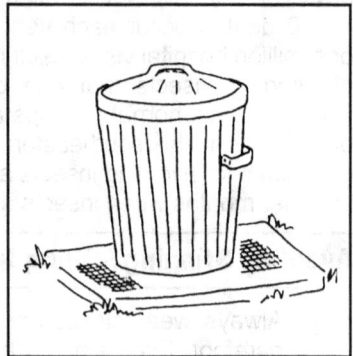

☞ Avoid consuming candies, popsicles, ice cream cones and soft drinks outdoors during warm weather. Stinging insects are attracted to sweets.

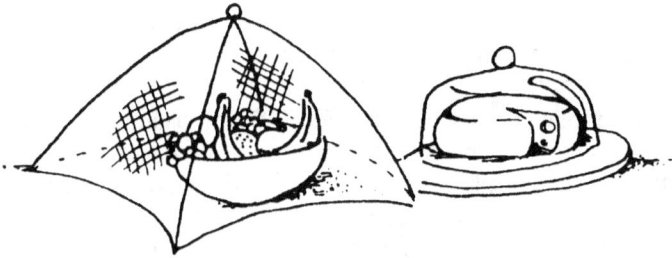

☞ If a bee or wasp lands on you, gently blow it away. Do not slap it or make rapid or jerking movements. If one flies into your car, open all windows, and it will probably fly out.

☞ Do not attempt to remove bees or wasps nests yourself. Always hire a professional exterminator.

☞ If you have been stung by a bee and the barbed stinger is left in the skin, to minimize more venom being injected into the skin, do the following: try to gently lift the stinger using a finger nail or knife edge to "flick" the stinger out of the skin. Do not pinch the stinger.

Avoiding Anaphylaxis from food

Ten foods are responsible for 90% of allergic reactions: peanuts, tree nuts (walnuts, cashews, almonds etc.), fish, shellfish, eggs, milk, soy, wheat, sesame seeds and sulfites. It is believed 3 million people in North America are allergic to peanuts. In North America between 6% - 8% of children and 1% - 3% of adults have food allergies.

To check if you or your child is allergic to certain food, as well as the skin or blood test already mentioned, there is another test called the elimination diet that your physician can do. The good news is that many children do "grow out" of their food allergies.

☞ Try to find out which foods you or your child is allergic to through your physician.

☞ The 100% effective avoidance measure is to avoid the allergenic food, which requires careful planning, research and vigilance.

☞ Find out if your food is a hidden ingredient within a meal. e.g. Peanut oil is used in Asian cooking, eggs can be in cookies and pastries.

☞ Check food labels. Since January 2006 manufacturers of foods, must list on their labels whether a food contains any of the eight most common food allergens.

☞ Avoidance can mean not actually touching the allergenic food and diligently washing your hands at appropriate times.

☞ Ensure cross contamination does not take place, where a utensil could have been used with a food allergen and used preparing your meal. Do not share utensils.

☞ Use caution in restaurants. Make sure the staff knows you are allergic to certain foods and ask about the ingredients within a meal.

☞ Make sure schools, caregivers, babysitters etc. understand what to do in case of an emergency. Complete the Anaphylaxis Action Plan like the example shown on the following page. This can be downloaded from the internet by going to www.twinject.com, clicking on CONSUMER, then on the left hand side clicking Anaphylaxis Action Plan.

Wearing MedicAlert®
Provides Peace of Mind

MedicAlert® "speaks" for people experiencing anaphylaxis who may have difficulty speaking or who are unconscious. Paramedics are trained to look for this immediately.

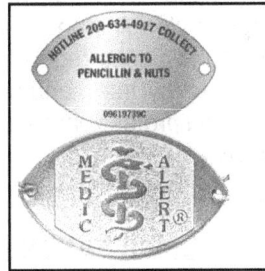

The MedicAlert® bracelet or necklace is engraved with the person's medical condition, membership number and the MedicAlert 24-hour Emergency Response Center telephone number. This Center can provide further medical information and also calls the members' emergency contacts. Phoning MedicAlert® at 1- 800-668-1507 can be a lifesaving preventative step to take.

HOME APPLIANCES THAT CAN HELP

It is important to keep the temperature and humidity in your home as constant as possible. Air that is very dry and areas that are damp are causes for concern. Check your thermostat to be sure that the temperature remains around 68 to 70 degrees Fahrenheit (20 to 21 degrees Centigrade). A hygrometer in the bedroom of the allergy sufferer can help monitor and maintain the humidity at an optimal level.

There are devices to heat, cool, humidify, dehumidify, and filter the air in your home. Some are expensive. Because of cost, it is in your interest to first implement the other measures described to control the environment in your home. However, in severe cases, these appliances can provide enormous relief to the allergy sufferer and are, therefore, worth the investment.

Whether these units are portable or built-in, they require regular cleaning and maintainence. Filters should be cleaned and/or replaced regularly, probably more often than is recommended by the manufacturer. Furnaces and ducts should be cleaned professionally once a year, preferably before the onset of winter.

VACUUM CLEANERS

The major problem with vacuum cleaners is that, although they pick up dust and larger particles, they blow out some of the house dust (the finer particles, including house dust mite debris). This can be worse for the allergy sufferer than not vacuuming! The use of a central vacuum, with an outside vent in the basement, ensures that no dust is recirculated. Easy-Flo® is recommended by *Consumer Reports*. An alternative is the use of a vacuum cleaner with a HEPA filtration system, such as Oreck®.

AIR PURIFIERS

An effective air purifier can really help sensitive individuals by providing a cleaner breathing environment. We stated in Chapter Four that the bedroom is a critical area in which to consider using an air purifier. However, it must be emphasized that an air purifier is not a substitute for the common-sense suggestions made in this booklet. The air purifier is a useful adjunct for eliminating pollutants and allergens.

Air purifiers work in several ways: there are mechanical filters that physically trap the particles; charcoal filters that absorb odors like cigarette smoke and cooking fumes; and electronic methods that remove particles from the air. Consult your physician or a reputable air purifier dealer to learn which air purifier suits your needs.

HEPA AIR PURIFIERS

Most physicians and respiratory organizations recommend the HEPA method of air filtration as the most effective. HEPA stands for High Efficiency Particulate Arresting.

HEPA air filtration is commonly used in hospital operating rooms. A clinical study of HEPA air purifiers was conducted in allergy patients' homes. Some machines had HEPA filters; others had blank filters. The results: patients who had HEPA filters in their homes had fewer symptoms and required less medication than those who had blank filters.

It is possible to obtain a tax refund on the purchase of HEPA air purifiers if the purchase is recommended by a physician.

FURNACE FILTERS

Nonelectrical Electrostatic Filters

These work similarly to the way electrostatic charges pick up small pieces of paper. These filters are made of a material that is positively and negatively charged. When air is forced through this material, pollen and dust are "zapped" out of the air. These filters are very efficient, require little maintainence (washed every two months), are easy to install, and remain effective for a long time. The filters do not use electricity and cost from $100 to $300.

Electronic Furnace Filters

Electronic furnace filters work similarly to the nonelectrical electrostatic furnace filters except that they use electricity to create the electrostatic charge. The Honeywell® F50E and the Trion Max® 5-1400 are recommended. These products cost over $1,000 each, require additional installation cost, and require electricity to operate. *Consumer Reports* rates electronic furnace filters as somewhat more effective than nonelectrical electrostatic filters.

AIR CONDITIONERS

Air conditioners remove particulates like dust, pollen, and mold spores from the air. Windows should be kept closed during periods when pollen counts are high. Clean the coils and filters regularly, and don't set the temperature controls too low. Air that is too cold aggravates breathing problems.

HUMIDIFIERS AND DEHUMIDIFIERS

These appliances can be the key to eliminating the mold and dust mite problems in your home. **Mites and mold proliferate in relative humidity of over 50%.** Humidity is the amount of moisture in the air; "relative humidity" is the percentage of the maximum amount of moisture air can hold at a given temperature. A dehumidifier draws indoor air over cooling coils by means of a fan. This condenses on the coil creating water droplets, which then drain into a bucket or floor drain. Better brands have adjustable humidistats so that you can set the optimum level of humidity. You have to choose the right capacity for your needs.

APPLIANCES TO CONSIDER

Central Vacuum System	❏
HEPA Vacuum Cleaner	❏
Air Purifier	❏
Furnace Filter	❏
Dehumidifier	❏
Air Conditioner	❏

CHAPTER SEVEN

THE IDEAL HOME ENVIRONMENT

I f you build your own home, and either you or a family member is an allergy or asthma sufferer, you have the opportunity to provide the optimal design for a more allergen-free and irritant-free environment.

GUIDELINES FOR THE IDEAL HOME ENVIRONMENT

☞ Install a central vacuum system to reduce the risk of recirculating dust. The collection container should be isolated and sealed.

☞ Design bedrooms in accordance with the guidelines in Chapter Four. For example, do not build closets in the allergy sufferer's bedroom.

☞ Avoid heating the house with a blower furnace; use electric or hot water heat.

☞ Avoid ceramic or vinyl tiles. Use sheet vinyl to avoid seams or crevices that collect dirt, mold, and dust.

☞ Install a central air-conditioning unit appropriate for the house.

☞ Keep garages and workshops as far away as possible from the house. If you want the garage attached to the house, do not position it below the bedrooms.

☞ Consult with the builder to ensure that all materials used, especially insulation materials, are allergen-free, if possible.

☞ Maintain clean lines throughout the house. Nooks and crannies are dust-catchers and create areas for insects to breed.

☞ Ensure that heat-generating appliances—refrigerators, televisions, radios, VCRs, DVD players, microwave ovens, ranges, and dishwashers—can be moved. The refrigerator base is a notorious harbor for food particles, insects, and dust.

☞ Doors and windows should be tight-fitting, with screens to prevent the entry of outdoor pollutants.

☞ Avoid tile floors in bathrooms; the grouting is hard to keep clean and encourages mold growth.

☞ The kitchen should have an exhaust fan that removes fumes, cooking odors, and smoke.

☞ Cement floors and walls of basements and cellars should be painted with paints that waterproof, retard mold growth, and inhibit dust formation.

☞ Recreation areas and living quarters should not be built below ground level to avoid dampness. Ideally, there should be no basement or cellar.

☞ The washing machine and clothes dryer should be in an enclosed room with the dryer vented outdoors. The furnace should be in a sealed area accessible from the outside.

☞ Avoid a lot of shrubbery around the house. Prune trees, hedges, and bushes regularly.

☞ The "mud room" should be separate from the living area, so that damp shoes, boots, galoshes, and sneakers can dry out.

☞ Garbage receptacles should be protected from animals and birds by placing them in a shed.

☞ Store food in a pantry that is easily checked for mold growth and insect infestation.

☞ Avoid carpeting. Choose instead wood floors or another easy-to-clean material. If you do have rugs, they should be washable.

☞ Carefully plan for a comprehensive approach to ensure optimum Indoor Air Quality (IAQ). It is important that all issues such as humidity (dehumidifier installation), furnace filter units, air conditioning, etc. collectively work in harmony.

Even if you can not build the "ideal" house, these guidelines can help you when you are in the market for a new home.

SYMPTOM ASSOCIATION DIARY

Complete the Symptom Association Diary for a week, a month, or a year. Record your symptoms, where you were and what you were doing when you experienced them, the weather conditions, and any strong odors. Record what you suspect to be the cause(s), but remember that your suspicions should be confirmed by your physician.

Rate the severity of your symptoms from 1 to 3, according to the following guidelines.

Level 1
Noticeable, but not debilitating

Level 2
Somewhat irritating, and a cause for concern

Level 3
Absorbing most of my thoughts.
Relief is a top priority!

*Photocopy the following diary for
whatever time period you require.*

Date/Time	Symptoms/Severity (1, 2, 3)	Location/Activity

Weather Conditions	Strong Odor(s)	Suspected Cause(s)

Ten Ways To
Help Yourself

This booklet contains a lot of information, so it is natural to feel a bit overwhelmed. These ten suggestions will help. Discuss your decisions with your doctor or pharmacist. Some measures will cost money, so evaluate their cost-effectiveness before you make a purchase.

1. **SEE YOUR DOCTOR.** Knowledge is power. You need to know what is causing your symptoms in order to avoid the causes and to discuss treatment options.

2. **COMPLY WITH YOUR TREATMENT.** Your physician may recommend allergy shots, or a non-drowsy antihistamine. Follow the recommended dosage listed in the packaging and follow the advice of your pharmacist..

3. **INSTALL A DEHUMIDIFIER.** To get to the root of the problem of mold and dust mite proliferation, ensure relative humidity is less than 50%. Mold and dust mites can be especially harmful to asthma patients as well as allergy sufferers.

4. **ALLERGY-PROOF BEDDING.** For those sensitive to house dust mites (especially asthma patients), clinical evidence proves this measure does help.

5. **PETS.** The only one hundred percent solution to the elimination of airborne dander is to remove the pet from the home. If this cannot be done, follow the suggestions in this book.

6. **EFFECTIVE VACUUMING.** Use a central vacuum system or a medically-approved vacuum cleaner, preferably one with a HEPA filter. The vacuum cleaner system must not recirculate the dust.

7. **BUY AN AIR PURIFIER.** This is especially important inthe bedroom.

8. **IMPROVE YOUR BEDROOM.** You spend a lot of time here. Make this room your "breathing oasis."

9. **IF YOU ARE AT RISK FOR ANAPHYLAXIS** . If you are allergic to insect stings, bites, foods or other allergens, make sure you carry a prescribed epinephrine injection such as TwinJect® and wear a Medic Alert® (1 800 668-1507) bracelet or necklet to inform people of your condition.

10. **READ THIS BOOKLET.** Take your time, take notes, and identify problem areas. Planning, thoroughness, and good maintenance habits are critical to success in allergy-proofing your home.

REMEMBER, KNOWLEDGE IS POWER.

CONCLUSION

There is no doubt that medical professionals recommend a "purer" home environment for allergy and asthma sufferers. Indeed, treatment can be enhanced by following the guidelines in this booklet. Your physician may have given or recommended it to you to help you create a healthier environment. However, compliance with all aspects of your treatment is the key to controlling your condition.

You are encouraged to analyze your symptoms and to link them to places and activities. Detective work is needed to uncover problem areas in your environment. The descriptions of the main offending allergens and irritants should give you a better understanding of "the enemies."

Perhaps one day there will be healthcare environmental consultants who will visit homes in order to develop efficient, cost-effective, allergen-free home environments. Until then, common sense, throughness, and effort on your part are vital.

USEFUL INFORMATION WEBSITES

Internet directory of allergy organizations and resources
www.allallergy.net

Allergy and Asthma Foundation of America (AAFA)
www.aafa.org

Allergy and Asthma Network Mothers of Asthmatics (AAN/ MA)
www.aanma.org

American Academy of Allergy, Asthma and Immunology (AAAAI)
www.aaaai.org

American College of Allergy, Asthma and Immunology (ACAAI)
www.allergy.mcg.edu

American Lung Association
www.lungusa.org

Allergy and Asthma Information
www.allergytreatment.net

National Air Duct Cleaners Association (NADCA) www.nadca.com
Pollen Counts www.pollen.com

Health House information - Lung Association
www.healthyhouse.org

Allergy Diagnosis: Hitachi Chemical Diagnostics
www.hcdiagnostics.com

Hydrasense
www.hydrasense.ca

MEDICAL INFORMATION

Astra Zeneca (Rhinocort ®)
www.astrazeneca.com
www.rhinocortni.com

Dey, L.P (Epipen®)
www.allergyreactions.com

Glaxo Smith Kline (Flonase®, Beconase AQ®)
www.asthmacontrol.com

MEDA Pharmaceuticals (Astelin®, Astepro®)
www.astelin.com
www.aboutrhinitis.com

Pfizer (Zyrtec®)
www.zyrtec.com/info

Sanofi-Aventis (Xyzal®, NaqsacortAQ®)
www.schering.com

Wyeth (Alavert®)
www.wyeth.com

OFFICIAL INFORMATION SERVICES

Consumer Products Safety
www.cpsc.gov/

Environmental Protection Agency
www.epa.gov

US Food and Drug Administration
www.da.gov/

Indoor Air Quality
www.epa.gov/iaq

National Asthma Education and Prevention Program
www.nhibi.nih.gov

National Institute of Allergy and Infectious Diseases
www.niaid.nih.gov/

National Institute for Occupational Safety and Health
www.cdc.gov/niosh

Hey Babysitter, Nanny, Caregiver, Teacher or Friend

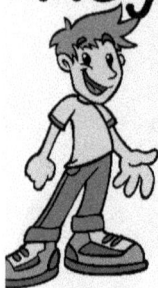

ASTHMA EMERGENCY ACTION PLAN

In case of a possible Severe Asthma Attack

Place child's photo here

Child's name:	Medic Alert #:
Nickname:	Home phone:
Address:	Cell phone:
Date of Birth:	Work phone:
Parent / guardian:	Emergency phone OR 911
Doctor's name:	Doctor's phone:

I Have No Asthma Symptoms.

I Have Asthma Symptoms, But I am in Control.

I Am In Danger and Need Help!

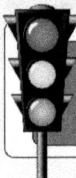

RED ZONE WARNING SYMPTOMS AND SIGNS

- Extreme cough, wheeze or chest tightness
- Shortness of breath, getting worse
- Difficulty walking or talking
- Hard time breathing
- Hunched over, struggling to breathe
- Reliever drug is not helping symptoms
- Peak flow meter reading is less than 60% of personal best
- Cannot perform usual activities
- Feeling faint and / or frightened
- Lips and fingernails are blue
- The attack came on suddenly

WHAT TO DO

1. **TELEPHONE 911** for emergency medical help and tell the dispatcher:
"A CHILD IS HAVING A LIFE THREATENING ASTHMA ATTACK."

2. **WHEN IN DOUBT** get to hospital emergency room as efficiently as possible.

OUR CHILD CAN HAVE AN ASTHMA ATTACK IF EXPOSED TO ANY OF THE FOLLOWING:

Tobacco Smoke · Dust Mites · Animals · Cockroaches · Outdoor grass, weed, tree pollen
· Molds · Strong Fumes · Exercise (when asthma not controlled)

☐ Peanuts ☐ Tree nuts ☐ Milk ☐ All dairy ☐ Eggs ☐ Shellfish ☐ Fish

Food additives (list)

Medications (list)

Others

OTHER EMERGENCY CONTACT INFORMATION

© 2007 Mediscript Communications Inc.

Asthma Emergency Action Poster
Available at your local pharmacy
or
email mediscript30@yahoo.ca
or visit:
www.mediscript.net or www.allergytreatment.net

www.ingramcontent.com/pod-product-compliance
Lightning Source LLC
Chambersburg PA
CBHW050601280326
41933CB00011B/1934